KIDNEY TRANSPLANT COOKBOOK

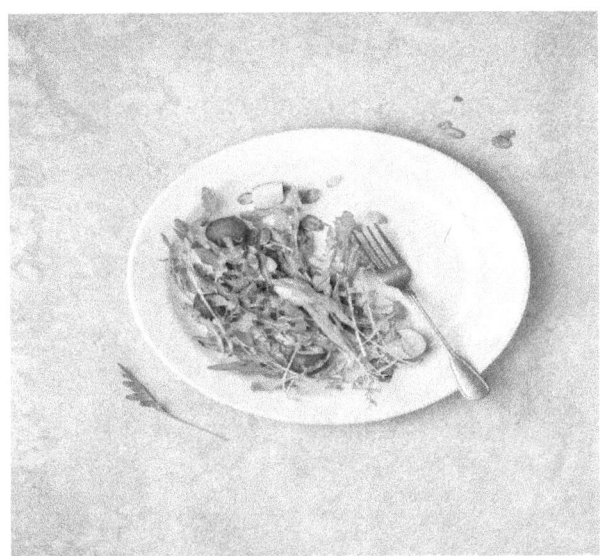

BENJAMIN THOMAS

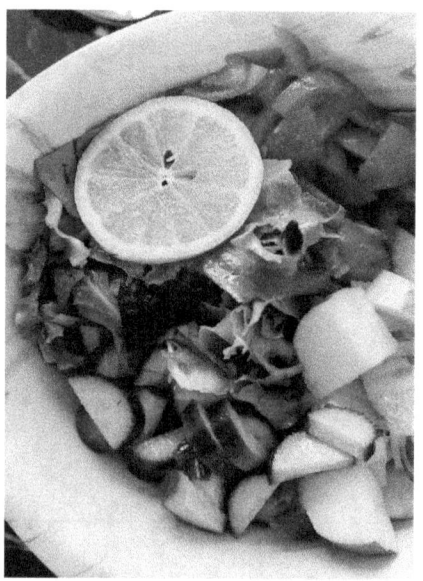

TABLE OF CONTENT

CHAPTER ONE 7

Introduction to Kidney Transplantation ...7

Overview of Kidney Transplant Process..9

Importance of Nutrition in Kidney Health
....12

Preparing for the Transplant Journey 15

Pre-transplant Dietary Guidelines 18

Symptoms of Kidney Transplant............21

CHAPTER TWO 23

Types of Kidney Transplant 23

Prevention of Kidney Transplant............24

Food to eat and avoid for kidney transplant
....27

CHAPTER THREE 31

Breakfast Kidney Transplant Recipes 31

1. Quinoa Breakfast Bowl: 31

2. Vegetable Omelette: 32

3. Greek Yogurt Parfait: 33

4. Sweet Potato and Spinach Breakfast Hash: 34

5. Chia Seed Pudding with Berries:........35

6. Banana-Oat Pancakes: 36

7. Cottage Cheese and Pineapple Parfait: 37

8. Egg and Veggie Breakfast Burrito: 37

9. Blueberry Almond Smoothie Bowl:...38

10. Spinach and Feta Breakfast Wrap: ...39

Lunch Kidney Transplant Recipes 40

1. Grilled Lemon Herb Chicken Salad: ..40

2. Quinoa and Roasted Vegetable Bowl:41

3. Salmon and Asparagus Foil Packets: .42

4. Mediterranean Chickpea Salad:.........43

5. Turkey and Avocado Wrap: 44

6. Vegetarian Lentil Soup:......................44

7. Eggplant and Tomato Stuffed Peppers:
....45

8. Tuna and White Bean Salad: 46

9. Shrimp Stir-Fry with Brown Rice: 47

10. Caprese Chicken Salad: 48

Dinner Kidney Transplant Recipes 49

1. Baked Lemon Herb Tilapia: 49

2. Vegetable and Chicken Skewers: 50

3. Spinach and Mushroom Stuffed Chicken
Breast: 51

4. Cauliflower and Chickpea Curry:........52

5. Lemon Garlic Shrimp Stir-Fry:..........52

6. Turkey and Vegetable Chili: 53

7. Roasted Vegetable and Quinoa Stuffed Peppers:.....................................54

8. Baked Herb-Crusted Cod: 55

9. Eggplant Lasagna: 56

10. Vegetarian Stir-Fried Rice:.............56

CONCLUSION 58

CHAPTER ONE

Introduction to Kidney Transplantation

Kidney transplantation is a life-changing medical procedure that offers renewed hope and vitality to individuals with end-stage renal disease (ESRD) or severe kidney dysfunction.

This transformative intervention involves the surgical transplantation of a healthy kidney from a living or deceased donor to a recipient whose own kidneys are no longer functioning adequately.

Understanding the intricacies of kidney transplantation is paramount for both patients and their caregivers, as it represents a crucial step towards reclaiming a fulfilling and healthier life.

The process of kidney transplantation begins with a thorough evaluation of the recipient's medical history, overall health, and compatibility with potential donors. Various factors, such as blood type, tissue matching, and the presence of antibodies, play a pivotal role in determining the suitability of a donor-recipient pair. Once a suitable match is identified, the transplant surgery is scheduled, marking the commencement of a transformative journey for the recipient.

For many individuals facing kidney failure, transplantation is often considered the most effective treatment option, providing a superior quality of life compared to long-term dialysis.

The benefits extend beyond improved physical health, encompassing psychological well-being and the restoration of a more normal daily routine.

While the prospect of kidney transplantation is promising, it comes with its own set of challenges and considerations. Post-transplant care involves a meticulous balance between the body's immune response and the need to prevent rejection of the transplanted organ.

Immunosuppressive medications, lifestyle adjustments, and vigilant monitoring become integral aspects of the recipient's ongoing healthcare regimen.

This introduction serves as a gateway to exploring the multifaceted landscape of kidney transplantation. From the initial stages of evaluation to the post-transplant care continuum, understanding the nuances of this medical procedure empowers individuals to actively participate in their healthcare journey, fostering resilience and optimism as they embark on the path to renewed health and vitality.

Overview of Kidney Transplant Process

The kidney transplant process is a complex yet meticulously orchestrated sequence of events designed to replace a failing or non-functioning kidney with a healthy organ, either from a living or deceased donor. This life-changing procedure offers a new lease on life for individuals grappling with end-stage renal disease

(ESRD) or severe kidney dysfunction, promising improved quality of life and enhanced overall well-being.

The journey typically begins with a comprehensive evaluation of both the potential recipient and potential donors.

A battery of tests assesses the medical compatibility, blood type, and tissue matching to ensure a successful transplant and minimize the risk of rejection.

The meticulous matching process aims to identify the most suitable donor-recipient pair, taking into account various immunological factors that may influence the likelihood of a positive outcome.

Once a suitable donor is identified, the transplant surgery is scheduled. Living donor transplants often provide a timelier option, as the surgery can be planned in advance.Deceased donor transplants, on the other hand, hinge on the availability of organs from individuals who have generously chosen to donate upon their passing. Timing is critical, and the transplant team works diligently to coordinate logistics and ensure the organ's viability for transplantation.

The surgical procedure itself involves the meticulous removal of the donor's kidney and its transplantation into the recipient. Advances in surgical techniques have led to minimally invasive procedures, reducing recovery times and postoperative discomfort.

Post-transplant, recipients undergo a period of close monitoring to detect and address any potential complications promptly.

To safeguard the transplanted organ from rejection, recipients' must adhere to a lifelong regimen of immunosuppressive medications.

Regular medical follow-ups, routine blood tests, and imaging studies are integral components of post-transplant care, ensuring the ongoing health and functionality of the transplanted kidney.

In essence, the kidney transplant process is a testament to medical advancements, teamwork, and the generosity of donors, offering a transformative solution for those grappling with kidney disease and ushering in a new chapter of vitality and improved health.

Importance of Nutrition in Kidney Health

Nutrition plays a pivotal role in maintaining kidney health, with its impact extending beyond basic sustenance to influencing the prevention and management of various kidney-related conditions.

The kidneys, essential organs for filtering waste and excess fluids from the blood, benefit significantly from a well-balanced and kidney-friendly diet.

Understanding the importance of nutrition in kidney health is fundamental for individual's at risk of kidney disease, those undergoing treatment, or those who have undergone a kidney transplant.

A kidney-friendly diet is designed to support optimal kidney function while mitigating the risk of complications. Managing the intake of key nutrients, such as sodium, potassium, phosphorus, and protein, becomes crucial in this regard.

Controlling sodium intake helps regulate blood pressure, reducing the strain on the kidneys. Meanwhile, monitoring potassium and phosphorus levels is essential to prevent imbalances that can adversely affect heart health and bone density.

For individuals with kidney disease, particularly those on dialysis, protein intake requires careful consideration. A balance must be struck to meet the body's needs while minimizing the burden on the kidneys.

Adequate protein is essential for muscle maintenance and overall health, but excessive protein consumption can lead to the accumulation of waste products that the impaired kidneys may struggle to eliminate.

Maintaining a healthy weight is another facet of kidney health that nutrition directly influences. Obesity and excess body weight are linked to an increased risk of developing kidney disease.

Adopting a nutrient-dense, portion-controlled diet, coupled with regular physical activity, contributes to weight management and overall well-being.

Post-kidney transplant, nutrition assumes a critical role in supporting the recovery process and ensuring the longevity of the transplanted organ. Balancing nutrient intake, staying hydrated, and adhering to dietary guidelines are essential components of post-transplant care.

In essence, the importance of nutrition in kidney health cannot be overstated. A well-informed and tailored approach to dietary choices empowers individuals to proactively manage their kidney health, reduce the risk of complications, and foster overall well-being. It serves as a cornerstone for a holistic approach to kidney care, complementing medical interventions and enhancing the potential for a healthier, more vibrant life.

Preparing for the Transplant Journey

The journey toward a kidney transplant is a significant chapter in the lives of individuals facing end-stage renal disease (ESRD) or severe kidney dysfunction. Adequate preparation for this transformative experience involves a combination of physical, emotional, and logistical considerations to optimize the likelihood of a successful outcome.

Medical Evaluations: A thorough medical evaluation is the initial step in preparing for a kidney transplant. Both potential recipients and living donors undergo a battery of tests to assess overall health, blood type, tissue compatibility, and the presence of antibodies.

This process ensures the identification of a suitable donor-recipient pair, minimizing the risk of rejection and complications during and after the transplant surgery.

Psychosocial Assessment: Beyond the physical aspects, psychosocial factors are also evaluated. Transplant teams assess the mental and emotional well-being of both recipients and donors, recognizing the importance of a strong support system and mental resilience throughout the transplant journey.

Pre-transplant Dietary Guidelines: Nutrition plays a critical role in preparing for a kidney transplant. Pre-transplant dietary guidelines may include restrictions on certain foods and adjustments to nutrient intake to optimize overall health and facilitate a smoother recovery post-transplant.

Coordination and Planning: For living donor transplants, coordination between the donor and recipient is crucial. This involves scheduling the transplant surgery at a time convenient for both parties, ensuring optimal conditions for the procedure.

In the case of deceased donor transplants, logistics related to organ procurement and transportation are carefully planned to minimize delays.

Education and Counseling: Education is a cornerstone of transplant preparation. Recipients and their families receive detailed information about the transplant process, post-transplant care, and potential lifestyle changes. Counseling services are often available to address concerns, alleviate anxiety, and provide emotional support.

Financial and Insurance Planning: The financial aspects of a kidney transplant can be substantial. Preparing for the transplant journey involves understanding insurance coverage, estimating out-of-pocket expenses, and exploring financial assistance options to alleviate the burden on the individuals involved.

By addressing these multifaceted aspects, individuals and their support networks can embark on the transplant journey with a comprehensive and well-prepared approach.

This preparation not only enhances the chances of a successful transplant but also contributes to a more seamless and positive experience for all parties involved.

Pre-transplant Dietary Guidelines

The period leading up to a kidney transplant is a critical phase that demands careful attention to dietary choices and lifestyle habits.

Pre-transplant dietary guidelines are designed to optimize the recipient's health, support overall well-being, and create an environment conducive to a successful transplant. Here are key considerations for individuals preparing for a kidney transplant:

Balanced Nutrition: A well-balanced diet is essential to maintain overall health and prepare the body for the challenges of surgery.

This includes a variety of fruits, vegetables, lean proteins, whole grains, and limited saturated fats. Adequate intake of essential nutrients supports the immune system and helps the body cope with the stress of surgery.

Limiting Sodium Intake: Sodium, found in salt, can contribute to high blood pressure and fluid retention, both of which can strain the kidneys.

Pre-transplant dietary guidelines often recommend limiting sodium intake to help manage blood pressure and reduce the risk of fluid buildup.

Fluid Management: Maintaining a proper fluid balance is crucial. While staying adequately hydrated is important, excessive fluid intake can lead to complications such as electrolyte imbalances. Pre-transplant guidelines may provide recommendations for daily fluid intake based on individual health status.

Protein Moderation: For individuals with kidney disease, especially those on dialysis, protein intake may be a consideration. While protein is essential for maintaining muscle mass and overall health, excessive protein consumption can burden the kidneys.

Pre-transplant dietary guidelines may include recommendations for moderate protein intake based on the individual's health status.

Avoiding Certain Foods: Depending on the individual's health condition, there may be specific dietary restrictions. For example, those with advanced kidney disease may be advised to limit potassium and phosphorus-rich foods. Pre-transplant dietary guidelines tailor recommendations to the unique needs of each patient.

Maintaining a Healthy Weight: Achieving and maintaining a healthy weight is crucial for overall well-being. Obesity can be a risk factor for complications during and after surgery. Pre-transplant dietary guidelines may include recommendations for weight management through portion control and a balanced diet.

Adhering to these pre-transplant dietary guidelines not only helps optimize the recipient's health but also contributes to the success of the transplant procedure.

These guidelines, often provided by a multidisciplinary transplant team, serve as an integral part of the comprehensive care plan, preparing individuals physically and nutritionally for the transformative journey ahead.

Symptoms of Kidney Transplant

Symptoms of kidney transplant primarily revolve around monitoring for potential complications or signs of rejection. In the initial weeks and months post-transplant, recipients are closely observed for any abnormal signs that might indicate issues with thetransplanted kidney or the body's response to it. Common symptoms include:

Swelling and Fluid Retention: Edema or swelling, especially in the extremities or around the eyes, can be an early sign of fluid retention, indicating potential issues with kidney function.

Changes in Urination: Paying attention to changes in urine output, color, or frequency is crucial.

Decreased urine output, dark urine, or changes in the pattern of urination can be indicative of kidney-related concerns.

Fatigue and Weakness: Persistent fatigue and weakness may suggest an imbalance or inadequate kidney function, leading to the accumulation of waste products in the body.

Fever and Infection: Elevated body temperature may indicate infection. Post-transplant, individuals are more susceptible to infections due to immunosuppressive medications.

Pain or Discomfort: Discomfort or pain around the transplant site or in the lower back could signal issues such as infection or rejection.

High Blood Pressure: Monitoring blood pressure is crucial, as hypertension can strain the kidneys and lead to complications.

It's important for transplant recipients to promptly report any unusual symptoms to their healthcare team.

CHAPTER TWO

Types of Kidney Transplant

There are two main types of kidney transplants: living donor transplants and deceased donor transplants.

Living Donor Transplants: In this type of transplant, a healthy individual voluntarily donates one of their kidneys to the recipient.

Living donor transplants offer several advantages, including better matching potential, the ability to plan the surgery in advance, and generally quicker recovery times for both the donor and the recipient.

The most common living donors are family members, but in some cases, close friends or unrelated individuals may also choose to donate.

Deceased Donor Transplants: Deceased donor transplants involve the use of kidneys from individuals who have passed away but have chosen to donate their organs. These kidneys are procured from deceased donors, typically individuals who have suffered brain death but still have viable organs. Deceased donor transplants rely on organ procurement organizations to match organs with recipients based on factors such as blood type, tissue compatibility, and medical urgency.

Both types of kidney transplants have their unique considerations, advantages, and challenges. The choice between living and deceased donor transplants often depends on the specific circumstances of the recipient, the availability of suitable donors, and the urgency of the transplant.

Prevention of Kidney Transplant

Prevention of kidney transplant refers to efforts aimed at preserving the health of the kidneys and minimizing the risk of kidney failure, thereby reducing the necessity for a transplant. Several strategies contribute to the prevention of kidney transplant:

Management of Underlying Conditions: Many cases of kidney disease stem from underlying health conditions such as diabetes and hypertension.

Controlling and managing these conditions through lifestyle modifications, medication adherence, and regular medical check-ups can significantly reduce the risk of kidney disease progression.

Healthy Lifestyle Choices: Adopting a healthy lifestyle, including a balanced diet low in salt and saturated fats, regular exercise, and maintaining a healthy weight, contributes to overall kidney health.

These practices help manage blood pressure, reduce the risk of diabetes, and prevent obesity-related kidney complications.

Hydration: Staying adequately hydrated is crucial for kidney function. Drinking an ample amount of water helps flush out toxins and waste products from the body, promoting optimal kidney health.

Avoiding Nephrotoxic Substances: Minimizing exposure to nephrotoxic substances such as certain medications, recreational drugs, and environmental toxins helps prevent damage to the kidneys.

Regular Health Check-ups: Routine health check-ups enable the early detection of potential kidney issues. Monitoring kidney function through blood tests, urinalysis, and blood pressure measurements allows for timely intervention and preventive measures.

Preventive Care in High-Risk Individuals: Individuals with a family history of kidney disease or those at higher risk due to conditions like polycystic kidney disease should undergo regular screenings and adopt preventive measures to minimize the risk of kidney-related complications.

Glomerulonephritis: Inflammation of the kidney's filtering units, known as glomeruli, can be caused by infections, immune system disorders, or other factors, leading to kidney damage.

Autoimmune Diseases: Conditions like lupus, where the immune system mistakenly attacks the body's own tissues, can affect the kidneys and contribute to kidney failure.

Infections: Severe and recurrent kidney infections can result in scarring and damage, eventually leading to kidney failure.

Understanding the underlying causes of kidney failure is crucial for determining the appropriate course of treatment, with kidney transplant being a viable option for many individuals with end-stage kidney disease.

Food to eat and avoid for kidney transplant

Maintaining a kidney-friendly diet is crucial for individuals who have undergone a kidney transplant. A balanced and mindful approach to nutrition can help support the health of the transplanted kidney and reduce the risk of complications. Here are guidelines on foods to eat and avoid:

Foods to Eat:

Low-Potassium Fruits and Vegetables: Opt for fruits and vegetables with lower potassium content, such as apples, berries, cauliflower, and green beans.

This helps manage potassium levels, as elevated levels can be problematic for kidney transplant recipients.

Lean Proteins: Choose lean protein sources like poultry, fish, eggs, and plant-based proteins such as tofu and legumes. Adequate protein intake is essential for muscle maintenance and overall health.

Whole Grains: Incorporate whole grains like brown rice, quinoa, and whole wheat bread. These provide fiber and essential nutrients without contributing excessive phosphorus.

Healthy Fats: Include sources of healthy fats, such as olive oil, avocados, and nuts, to support overall heart and kidney health.

Low-Sodium Options: Limit sodium intake by choosing fresh, whole foods and using herbs and spices for flavoring instead of salt. Excessive sodium can contribute to high blood pressure and fluid retention.

Calcium-Rich Foods: Consume adequate calcium from sources like low-fat dairy products, fortified plant-based milk, and leafy green vegetables. Calcium is essential for bone health, especially for individuals on immunosuppressive medications.

Foods to Avoid:

High-Potassium Foods: Minimize high-potassium foods like bananas, oranges, tomatoes, and potatoes, as they can contribute to elevated potassium levels.

Phosphorus-Rich Foods: Limit phosphorus intake by avoiding processed foods, colas, and high-phosphorus foods like dairy products, nuts, and certain beans.

High-Sodium Foods: Reduce the consumption of processed and salty foods, including canned soups, deli meats, and fast food, to manage blood pressure and prevent fluid retention.

Excessive Protein: While protein is essential, excessive intake can strain the kidneys. Work with a healthcare professional to determine the appropriate amount for your individual needs.

Alcohol and Caffeine: Limit alcohol intake and monitor caffeine consumption, as both can affect hydration and potentially interact with medications.

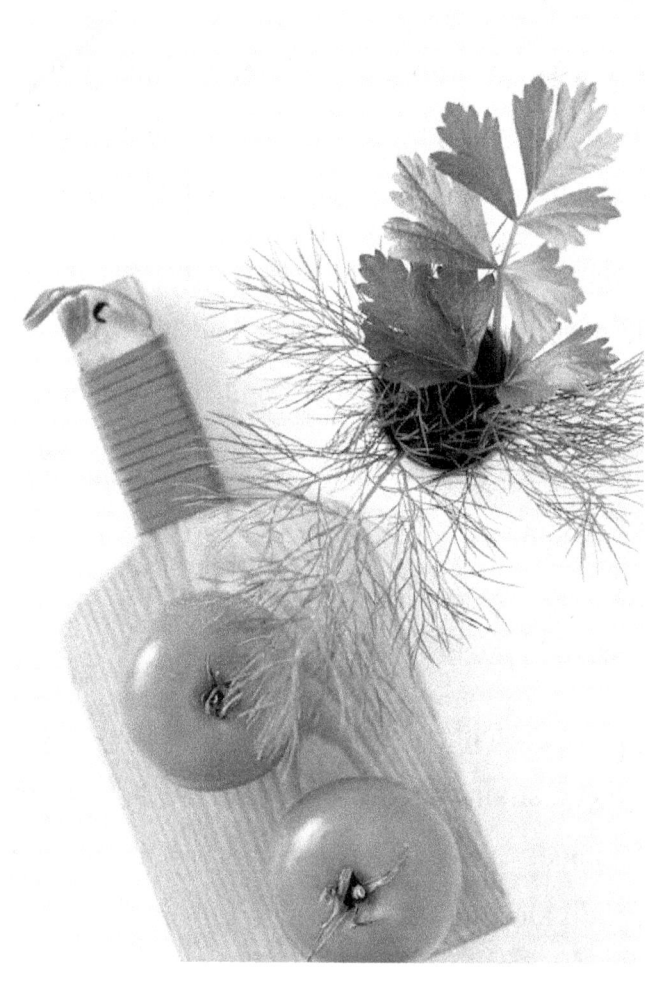

CHAPTER THREE

Breakfast Kidney Transplant Recipes

1. Quinoa Breakfast Bowl:

Ingredients:

- 1/2 cup cooked quinoa
- 1/4 cup diced strawberries
- 1/4 cup blueberries
- 1 tablespoon chopped almonds
- 1 tablespoon honey

Instructions:

- In a bowl, combine cooked quinoa, strawberries, blueberries, and chopped almonds.
- Drizzle with honey for added sweetness.
- Mix well and enjoy a protein-packed, nutrient-rich breakfast.

Preparation Time: 10 minutes

2. Vegetable Omelette:

Ingredients:

- 2 large eggs
- 1/4 cup diced bell peppers
- 1/4 cup chopped spinach
- 1 tablespoon feta cheese (optional)
- Salt and pepper to taste

Instructions:

- Whisk eggs in a bowl and season with salt and pepper.
- Stir in bell peppers and spinach.
- Pour the mixture into a heated, non-stick skillet.
- Cook until the eggs are set, folding the omelette in half.
- Sprinkle with feta cheese if desired and serve.

Preparation Time: 15 minute

3. Greek Yogurt Parfait:

Ingredients:

- 1/2 cup Greek yogurt
- 1/4 cup granola (low phosphorus)
- 1/4 cup sliced peaches
- 1 tablespoon chia seeds

Instructions:

- In a glass or bowl, layer Greek yogurt, granola, and sliced peaches.
- Sprinkle chia seeds on top for added texture and nutrition.
- Repeat layers and serve this delicious and protein-rich parfait.

Preparation Time: 5 minutes

4. Sweet Potato and Spinach Breakfast Hash:

Ingredients:

- 1 small sweet potato, peeled and diced
- 1/2 cup diced onions
- 1 cup chopped spinach
- 1 tablespoon olive oil
- 2 eggs (optional)

Instructions:

- In a skillet, heat olive oil and sauté onions until translucent.
- Add diced sweet potatoes and cook until tender.
- Stir in chopped spinach until wilted.
- Optionally, serve with a poached or fried egg on top for extra protein.

Preparation Time: 20 minutes

5. Chia Seed Pudding with Berries:

Ingredients:

- 2 tablespoons chia seeds
- 1/2 cup almond milk (unsweetened)
- 1/4 teaspoon vanilla extract
- 1/2 cup mixed berries (blueberries, raspberries, strawberries)
- 1 tablespoon chopped walnuts (optional)

Instructions:

- In a bowl, mix chia seeds, almond milk, and vanilla extract. Stir well and refrigerate overnight.
- In the morning, top the chia pudding with mixed berries and chopped walnuts.
- Enjoy a nutrient-dense and fiber-rich breakfast.

Preparation Time: 5 minutes (plus overnight refrigeration)

6. Banana-Oat Pancakes:

Ingredients:

- 1 ripe banana, mashed
- 1/2 cup old-fashioned oats
- 1/4 cup milk (or non-dairy alternative)
- 1/2 teaspoon cinnamon
- 1 tablespoon chopped almonds

Instructions:

- In a bowl, mix mashed banana, oats, milk, and cinnamon to form a batter.
- Heat a non-stick skillet and spoon the batter to make small pancakes.
- Cook until edges are set, flip, and cook the other side.
- Sprinkle with chopped almonds and serve with a dollop of Greek yogurt if desired.

Preparation Time: 15 minutes

7. Cottage Cheese and Pineapple Parfait:

Ingredients:

- 1/2 cup low-fat cottage cheese
- 1/2 cup fresh pineapple chunks
- 1 tablespoon shredded coconut
- 1 tablespoon honey

Instructions:

- In a glass, layer cottage cheese, pineapple chunks, and shredded coconut.
- Drizzle with honey for added sweetness.
- Repeat layers and enjoy a protein-rich and tropical-flavored parfait.

Preparation Time: 10 minutes

8. Egg and Veggie Breakfast Burrito:

Ingredients:

- 1 whole wheat tortilla

- 2 large eggs, scrambled
- 1/4 cup diced tomatoes
- 1/4 cup chopped bell peppers
- 2 tablespoons shredded low-fat cheese

Instructions:

- In a skillet, cook scrambled eggs, diced tomatoes, and chopped bell peppers.
- Place the egg mixture on a whole wheat tortilla, sprinkle with shredded cheese, and roll into a burrito.
- Optional: Serve with a side of salsa for extra flavor.

Preparation Time: 15 minutes

9. Blueberry Almond Smoothie Bowl:

Ingredients:

- 1/2 cup frozen blueberries
- 1/2 banana
- 1/2 cup almond milk (unsweetened)

- 1 tablespoon almond butter
- Toppings: sliced almonds, chia seeds, fresh blueberries

Instructions:

- Blend frozen blueberries, banana, almond milk, and almond butter until smooth.
- Pour the smoothie into a bowl and add sliced almonds, chia seeds, and fresh blueberries as toppings.
- Enjoy a refreshing and nutrient-packed smoothie bowl.

Preparation Time: 5 minutes

10. Spinach and Feta Breakfast Wrap:

Ingredients:

- 1 whole grain wrap
- 2 eggs, scrambled
- 1/2 cup fresh spinach, chopped

- 2 tablespoons crumbled feta cheese
- Salt and pepper to taste

Instructions:

- In a skillet, cook scrambled eggs with chopped spinach until eggs are set.
- Place the egg and spinach mixture onto a whole grain wrap.
- Sprinkle with crumbled feta cheese and season with salt and pepper.
- Roll into a wrap and enjoy a protein and fiber-rich breakfast.

Preparation Time: 10 minutes

Lunch Kidney Transplant Recipes

1. Grilled Lemon Herb Chicken Salad:

Ingredients:

- 1 boneless, skinless chicken breast
- Mixed salad greens
- Cherry tomatoes, halved

- Cucumber, sliced
- Lemon vinaigrette (olive oil, lemon juice, herbs)

Instructions:

- Grill the chicken breast until fully cooked.
- Slice the chicken and arrange it on a bed of mixed salad greens.
- Add cherry tomatoes and cucumber slices.
- Drizzle with homemade lemon vinaigrette.

Preparation Time: 20 minutes

2. Quinoa and Roasted Vegetable Bowl:

Ingredients:

- 1/2 cup cooked quinoa
- Roasted vegetables (bell peppers, zucchini, eggplant)
- Chickpeas (canned, rinsed)
- Feta cheese (optional)
- Balsamic vinaigrette

Instructions:

- Combine cooked quinoa, roasted vegetables, and chickpeas in a bowl.
- Top with crumbled feta cheese if desired.
- Drizzle with balsamic vinaigrette.

Preparation Time: 25 minutes

3. Salmon and Asparagus Foil Packets:

Ingredients:

- Salmon fillet
- Asparagus spears
- Lemon slices
- Garlic, minced
- Olive oil

Instructions:

- Place salmon fillet and asparagus on a piece of foil.
- Top with lemon slices and minced garlic.

- Drizzle with olive oil, seal the foil packet, and bake until salmon is cooked.

Preparation Time: 30 minutes

4. Mediterranean Chickpea Salad:

Ingredients:

- Canned chickpeas, drained and rinsed
- Cherry tomatoes, halved
- Cucumber, diced
- Red onion, finely chopped
- Kalamata olives, sliced
- Feta cheese, crumbled
- Olive oil and lemon dressing

Instructions:

- Combine chickpeas, cherry tomatoes, cucumber, red onion, olives, and feta cheese in a bowl.
- Toss with olive oil and lemon dressing.

Preparation Time: 15 minutes

5. Turkey and Avocado Wrap:

Ingredients:

- Sliced turkey breast
- Whole wheat wrap
- Avocado, sliced
- Lettuce leaves
- Tomato slices

Instructions:

- Lay out a whole wheat wrap and layer with turkey slices.
- Add avocado slices, lettuce leaves, and tomato slices.
- Roll into a wrap and secure with toothpicks if needed.

Preparation Time: 10 minutes

6. Vegetarian Lentil Soup:

Ingredients:

- Dry lentils, rinsed

- Carrots, diced
- Celery, chopped
- Onion, diced
- Vegetable broth
- Garlic, minced
- Cumin, coriander, and turmeric (spices)

Instructions:

1. Combine lentils, carrots, celery, onion, garlic, and spices in a pot with vegetable broth.
2. Simmer until lentils and vegetables are tender.

Preparation Time: 40 minutes

7. Eggplant and Tomato Stuffed Peppers:

Ingredients:

- Bell peppers, halved
- Eggplant, diced
- Tomatoes, chopped
- Quinoa, cooked

- Feta cheese (optional)
- Italian seasoning

Instructions:

- Roast bell peppers until slightly tender.
- In a bowl, mix diced eggplant, chopped tomatoes, and cooked quinoa.
- Spoon the mixture into the bell pepper halves.
- Sprinkle with feta cheese and Italian seasoning.

Preparation Time: 35 minutes

8. Tuna and White Bean Salad:

Ingredients:

- Canned tuna, drained
- Cannellini beans, rinsed
- Red onion, finely chopped
- Parsley, chopped
- Lemon juice
- Olive oil

Instructions:

- In a bowl, combine tuna, cannellini beans, red onion, and parsley.
- Dress with lemon juice and olive oil.

Preparation Time: 15 minutes

9. Shrimp Stir-Fry with Brown Rice:

Ingredients:

- Shrimp, peeled and deveined
- Mixed vegetables (broccoli, bell peppers, snap peas)
- Brown rice, cooked
- Soy sauce
- Ginger and garlic, minced

Instructions:

- Stir-fry shrimp and mixed vegetables in a wok or skillet.
- Add minced ginger and garlic.

- Serve over cooked brown rice, drizzled with soy sauce.

Preparation Time: 25 minutes

10. Caprese Chicken Salad:

Ingredients:

- Grilled chicken breast, sliced
- Mixed salad greens
- Cherry tomatoes, halved
- Fresh mozzarella, sliced
- Basil leaves
- Balsamic glaze

Instructions:

- Arrange sliced grilled chicken on a bed of mixed salad greens.
- Add cherry tomatoes, fresh mozzarella slices, and basil leaves.
- Drizzle with balsamic glaze.

Preparation Time: 20 minutes

Dinner Kidney Transplant Recipes

1. Baked Lemon Herb Tilapia:

Ingredients:

- Tilapia fillets
- Lemon juice
- Fresh herbs (rosemary, thyme)
- Olive oil
- Garlic, minced

Instructions:

- Preheat the oven and place tilapia fillets on a baking sheet.
- Mix lemon juice, fresh herbs, olive oil, and minced garlic to make a marinade.
- Pour the marinade over the tilapia and bake until the fish flakes easily.

Preparation Time: 25 minutes

2. Vegetable and Chicken Skewers:

Ingredients:

- Chicken breast, cut into cubes
- Bell peppers (assorted colors), cut into chunks
- Cherry tomatoes
- Red onion, cut into wedges
- Olive oil and balsamic vinegar

Instructions:

- Thread chicken cubes and vegetables onto skewers.
- Brush with a mixture of olive oil and balsamic vinegar.
- Grill or bake until chicken is cooked through.

Preparation Time: 30 minutes

3. Spinach and Mushroom Stuffed Chicken Breast:

Ingredients:

- Chicken breasts
- Fresh spinach
- Mushrooms, chopped
- Garlic, minced
- Feta cheese (optional)

Instructions:

- Preheat the oven and butterfly chicken breasts.
- Sauté spinach, mushrooms, and garlic until wilted.
- Fill each chicken breast with the spinach-mushroom mixture and bake.
- Optionally, sprinkle with feta cheese before serving.

Preparation Time: 40 minutes

4. Cauliflower and Chickpea Curry:

Ingredients:

- Cauliflower florets
- Canned chickpeas, drained
- Onion, chopped
- Garlic and ginger, minced
- Curry spices (turmeric, cumin, coriander)
- Coconut milk

Instructions:

- Sauté onion, garlic, and ginger until softened.
- Add cauliflower, chickpeas, and curry spices. Stir well.
- Pour in coconut milk and simmer until cauliflower is tender.

Preparation Time: 35 minutes

5. Lemon Garlic Shrimp Stir-Fry:

Ingredients:

- Shrimp, peeled and deveined

- Broccoli florets
- Bell peppers, sliced
- Snow peas
- Lemon juice
- Soy sauce

Instructions:

- Stir-fry shrimp and vegetables in a wok or skillet.
- Add lemon juice and soy sauce for flavor.
- Serve over brown rice or quinoa.

Preparation Time: 20 minutes

6. Turkey and Vegetable Chili:

Ingredients:

- Ground turkey
- Kidney beans, drained and rinsed
- Diced tomatoes
- Bell peppers, diced
- Onion, chopped
- Chili powder and cumin

Instructions:

- Brown ground turkey in a pot with diced onion.
- Add kidney beans, diced tomatoes, bell peppers and spices.
- Simmer until flavors meld together.

Preparation Time: 45 minutes

7. Roasted Vegetable and Quinoa Stuffed Peppers:

Ingredients:

- Quinoa, cooked
- Mixed roasted vegetables (zucchini, cherry tomatoes, bell peppers)
- Feta cheese (optional)
- Fresh basil, chopped

Instructions:

- Combine cooked quinoa, roasted vegetables, and feta cheese in a bowl.
- Stuff bell peppers with the quinoa mixture.

- Bake until peppers are tender.

Preparation Time: 30 minutes

8. Baked Herb-Crusted Cod:

Ingredients:

- Cod fillets
- Bread crumbs
- Fresh herbs (parsley, dill)
- Lemon zest
- Olive oil

Instructions:

- Preheat the oven and place cod fillets on a baking sheet.
- Mix bread crumbs, fresh herbs, lemon zest, and olive oil to create a crust.
- Press the crust onto the cod fillets and bake until golden.

Preparation Time: 25 minutes

9. Eggplant Lasagna:

Ingredients:

- Eggplant, thinly sliced
- Ground turkey or beef
- Tomato sauce
- Ricotta cheese
- Mozzarella cheese, shredded

Instructions:

- Grill or bake eggplant slices until tender.
- In a baking dish, layer eggplant, ground meat, tomato sauce, and cheeses.
- Repeat layers and bake until bubbly.

Preparation Time: 50 minutes

10. Vegetarian Stir-Fried Rice:

Ingredients:

- Brown rice, cooked
- Mixed vegetables (peas, carrots, corn)

- Tofu, diced
- Soy sauce
- Sesame oil

Instructions:

- Stir-fry tofu and mixed vegetables in a wok or skillet.
- Add cooked brown rice, soy sauce, and sesame oil.
- Cook until everything is heated through.

Preparation Time: 25 minutes

CONCLUSION

In concluding this kidney transplant cookbook, my utmost aim has been to provide a valuable resource for individuals on the transformative journey of kidney transplantation.

Nourishing your body with the right foods is not just a culinary endeavor but a profound investment in your well-being. Each recipe, guideline, and insight shared here aspires to empower you in embracing a kidney-friendly lifestyle, ensuring a harmonious post-transplant experience.

Remember, your kitchen is a sanctuary where healing ingredients can manifest into delectable creations. May this cookbook serve as a companion, offering both comfort and inspiration on your path to vibrant health after a kidney transplant.